NATURAL HOME REMEDIES

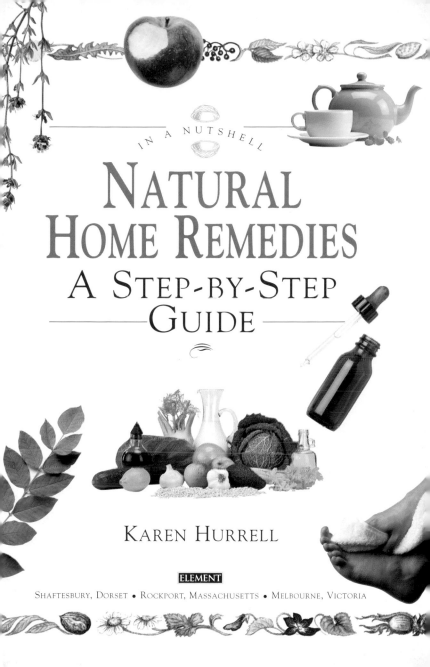

IN A NUTSHELL

NATURAL
HOME REMEDIES
A STEP-BY-STEP
GUIDE

KAREN HURRELL

ELEMENT

SHAFTESBURY, DORSET • ROCKPORT, MASSACHUSETTS • MELBOURNE, VICTORIA

© Element Books Limited 1997

First published
in Great Britain in
1997 by
ELEMENT BOOKS LIMITED
Shaftesbury,
Dorset, SP7 9BP

Published in the USA in 1997 by
ELEMENT BOOKS INC
PO Box 830, Rockport, MA 01966

Published in Australia in 1997 by
ELEMENT BOOKS LIMITED
and distributed by Penguin Australia Ltd
487 Maroondah Highway, Ringwood,
Victoria 3134

NOTE FROM THE PUBLISHER
Any information given in this
book is not intended to be taken
as a replacement for medical
advice. Any person with a condition
requiring medical attention should consult a
qualified practitioner or therapist.

*Designed and created with
The Bridgewater Book Company Ltd*

ELEMENT BOOKS LIMITED
Editorial Director Julia McCutchen
Managing Editor Caro Ness
Project Editor Allie West
Production Director Roger Lane
Production Sarah Golden

THE BRIDGEWATER BOOK COMPANY
Art Director Kevin Knight
Designers Andrew Milne, Jane Lanaway
Managing Editor Anne Townley
Project co-ordinator Fiona Corbridge
Page layout Chris Lanaway
Picture Research Lynda Marshall
Three dimensional models Mark Jamieson
Photography Ian Parsons, Guy Ryecart
Illustrations Andrew Milne, Pip Adams

Text consultants BOOK CREATION SERVICES LTD
Series Editor Karen Sullivan

Printed and bound by Dai Nippon, Hong Kong

British Library Cataloguing in
Publication data available

Library of Congress Cataloging
in Publication data available

ISBN 1-86204-108-3

*The publishers wish to thank the following for the
use of pictures:* Bridgeman Art Library, e.t.
archive, and Science Photo Library.

Special thanks go to:
Paul Castle, Natasha Gray, and
Jo Mortimer, *for help with
photography*

Contents

Introduction to natural medicine

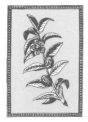

ABOVE **Nutmeg, from Mattioli's** Commentaires, *a 16th century herbal.*

FROM THE VERY *earliest times, people have exploited plants for their medicinal properties. Although our culture has welcomed the advent of modern medicine and its many benefits, the tradition of folk medicine and home remedies has kept its niche.*

Today, there is a new understanding of ecology and a greater concern about the side-effects of drugs, and there has been a remarkable resurgence in the use of natural medicine. In the past, every family had a wealth of favorite home remedies

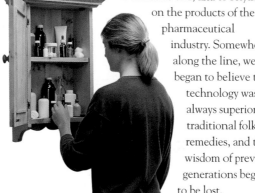

RIGHT **We have become accustomed to relying on the products of the pharmaceutical industry.**

that could be prepared to treat minor medical emergencies. Often, the treatment could be found in the garden or in the kitchen larder.

Modern medicine has led to a dependency on physicians. We have become accustomed to putting our health in the hands of someone else, and to relying on the products of the pharmaceutical industry. Somewhere along the line, we began to believe that technology was always superior to traditional folk remedies, and the wisdom of previous generations began to be lost.

Increasingly, however, we are learning that the conventional medical system is not infallible. These "miracle cures" may make us feel better, but all too many do so by suppressing the symptoms, not curing their cause. In the West, we are accustomed to taking medicine only when we are ill, and it is difficult to teach ourselves that good health means adopting a holistic approach. Natural remedies are designed to be holistic, considering the mind, body, and spirit as equally important elements of good health. When all three are balanced, when we have optimum energy levels and a good sense of well-being, our bodies will have the best chance of curing themselves.

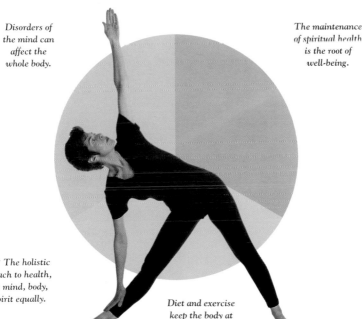

Disorders of the mind can affect the whole body.

The maintenance of spiritual health is the root of well-being.

RIGHT *The holistic approach to health, values mind, body, and spirit equally.*

Diet and exercise keep the body at optimum fitness.

A history of healing

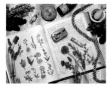

ABOVE **Many modern medicines are derived from the plants listed in early herbals.**

THE PRACTICE of using natural substances to treat and prevent illness has existed since prehistoric times, and is used today by up to 80 per cent of the world's population as a primary form of medicine. Many modern medicines come from plants, including aspirin from willow bark (Salix species) and digitalis from foxglove (Digitalis purpurea).

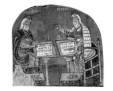

HIPPOCRATES AND GALEN

The chart shows the development of natural medicine from ancient times to the present day.

China	India	Egypt	Greece	Europe
Emperor Shen Nung's *Canon of Herbs* was the first authoritative chronicle of its type. During the Ming Dynasty, Li Shizhen compiled the world-famous *Materia Medica*, which was completed in 1578.	In India, since 2000 B.C.F. the advancement of medical and surgical skills included the use of hundreds of herbs, many of which are still used today.	*Papyrus Ebers* (published in the 1600 B.C.E.) names more than 700 herbal remedies. Egyptian physicians worked with nearly 1,000 herbs.	In the classical world, the father of medicine, Hippocrates (460–370 B.C.E.), refers to 300 medicinal plants in his works. Other medical authorities described the use of medical botany.	The Renaissance saw the development of natural medicine. Nicholas Culpeper translated the entire physicians' pharmacopoeia, *The English Physician and Complete Herbals*, in 1653.

ANIMAL HEALTH

Plants have always played a role in healing. Even animals use herbs for health – for example, blackbirds seek out berries in the winter months, to build up their iron and vitamin stores, and cats chew grass as a digestive when fur builds up in their guts. There is an extraordinary history of herbal healing for both human and beast, and it has been recorded from the beginning of time.

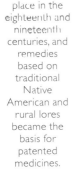

GATHERING SAGE

CULPEPPER

HERBALISM

Plants can often be used in preventive medicine – to balance and cleanse – and in the treatment of illness. In your garden, window box, larder, or in the countryside you will find an extensive personal and natural home medicine chest for preventative health measures, first aid, and normal everyday health needs. What you can't grow or pick yourself, you can purchase at a reputable herbalist or health shop.

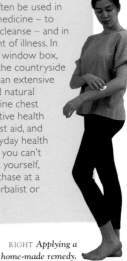

RIGHT *Applying a home-made remedy.*

USA

A revival of herbalism took place in the eighteenth and nineteenth centuries, and remedies based on traditional Native American and rural lores became the basis for patented medicines.

20th cent.

The use of herbs become less popular in the twentieth century, with the advent of orthodox medicine and the growing dependency on medical drugs. People grew to rely upon their physicians to find a cure for their sickness.

Pharmacy

The ability to synthesize plant parts called an end to the widespread use of natural herbs, and pharmaceutical companies encouraged a belief in the greater effectiveness of their drugs.

Today

As research into the active constituents of herbs continues, increasing numbers of ancient treatments and tonics are becoming recognized once more, and brought back into widespread use.

Side-effects

Growing concern about the side-effects of drugs, including the shocking tragedies with compounds such as thalidomide, has meant that natural medicine has experienced something of a renaissance.

Setting the scene

WHAT MAKES *up home remedies? The earth supplies us with a rich array of remedies to treat ailments of every type. We can find these remedies in our gardens, window boxes, larders, or in the fields. Today many shops also specialize in these products.*

THYME

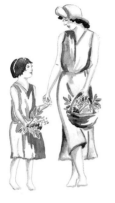

GATHERING HERBS AND PLANTS

Herbs, plants, foodstuffs, minerals, fruits and vegetables form the basis of both orthodox and traditional medicine. Their active ingredients are isolated to help produce modern drugs, but, best of all, they can be used naturally in many therapeutic forms, including flower essences, essential oils, homeopathic and herbal remedies.

FLOWER ESSENCE

LAVENDER

LEFT, ABOVE, AND RIGHT
The natural world provides a wealth of ingredients useful to the dedicated natural remedy practitioner.

HERBS AND PLANTS

In medicine, the term "herb" includes any plant, and any part of a plant, that can be used to make a remedy. This can include seaweeds, ferns, flowers, roots, bulbs, barks, seeds, and leaves. It includes cooking herbs, spices, and many fruits and vegetables.

Herbs are normally chosen to work with the inherent healing powers of the body. Many herbs strengthen and encourage the action of particular organs. Herbs are ideal medicines to use in the home for the treatment of both minor ailments and chronic diseases.

HOMEOPATHIC REME

FOODSTUFFS

Items in our larders have traditionally been used for medicinal purposes. Foodstuffs such as bread, cabbage, milk, yogurt, and vinegar have both nutritional properties, which can enhance health and prevent illness, and medicinal qualities, that allow them to treat specific conditions and prevent their recurrence. The benefit of foodstuffs is that they are normally easy to buy or prepare, and are ideal for those who prefer not to use prescription drugs or strong herbal preparations. Many of these items have a long history of traditional use.

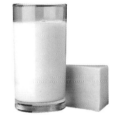
FRUIT

THERAPEUTIC FOODSTUFFS

ABOVE, LEFT AND RIGHT
You will already have a selection of therapeutic foodstuffs in your kitchen.

BREAD

MILK AND CHEESE

PURCHASING REMEDIES

Most herbs can be purchased already prepared, with dosage instructions included on the packaging. Homeopathic remedies – that is, those prepared according to the principles of homeopathy and diluted to create a useful remedy (such as flower essences, teas, and tinctures) – are all available at good health shops.

Many people enjoy making the remedies themselves, and it is often considered an important part of the healing process.

LEFT *Your local health shop will offer a wide range of herbal and homeopathic remedies.*

Preparing the remedies

PESTLE AND MORTAR

MANY PLANTS *and herbs need to be prepared to release active ingredients, or to convert them into a more useful form. For example, woody herbs must be boiled and "decocted" to make a tincture or drink.*

If you are suffering from a chronic or life-threatening condition, or you have an undiagnosed problem, it is wise to consult your physician or health practitioner (registered herbalist or homeopath) before treating yourself.

TINCTURES

Powdered, fresh, or dried herbs are placed in an air-tight container with alcohol and left for a period of time.

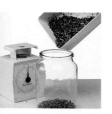

1 *You can make your own tincture by crushing plant parts (about 1oz/25g) and suspending them in alcohol (about 20fl oz/600ml of any 40 per cent spirit) for about two weeks, shaking occasionally. For dried herbs use 4oz/100g with the same amount of alcohol.*

2 *After straining, the liquid or tincture should be stored in a dark glass air-tight jar. Dosages are normally 5–20 drops, which can be taken directly or added to water.*

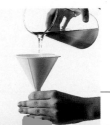

DECOCTIONS

The roots, twigs, berries, seeds, or bark of a plant are used. The
method is similar to that used to make an infusion.

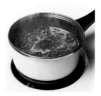

*2 The liquid is strained and
drunk with a bit of honey or
brown sugar, as often as
has been prescribed. Decoctions
should be refrigerated, and will
last about three days.*

*1 Boil the plant parts in water
to extract the ingredients.*

INFUSIONS

Effectively another word for tea, an infusion is made from dried
herbs, or in some instances fresh herbs, which are steeped in
boiling water for about ten minutes.

*1 Keep the lid on the teapot and
always use the purest water
available, to ensure that the
medicinal properties of the plant
are effectively obtained. You can
make herbal teabags
by cutting a rectangle
of muslin, fold, and
sew up the sides. Fill
with herbs and sew
across the top.*

*2 Strain the
infusion and
drink hot or cold,
either sweetened or
unsweetened.
Infusions should be made fresh
each day, if possible. Leaves and
flowers are best taken as
infusions, since their properties
are more easily extracted by
gentle boiling.*

TISANES

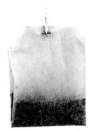

Tisanes are mild infusions, normally prepackaged and sold in the form of a teabag, which can be steeped for a much shorter period of time

HERBAL TEABAG

than an infusion. The chamomile tea available from supermarkets would be considered a tisane.

POWDERS

Powdered herbs can be added to food or drinks as they are, or put into capsules for easier consumption. You can make your own powder by crushing dried plant parts with a pestle and mortar, or chop them finely in a food processor or coffee grinder.

PILLS

HERBAL PILLS
AND CAPSULES

Herbal remedies are less common in pill form, as they are more difficult to produce. The more common remedies are available from health food shops, or you can press your own with a domestic press.

COMPRESSES AND POULTICES

Compresses and poultices are for external use and can be extremely effective since the active parts of the herb are able to reach the affected area without being altered in any way by the digestive tract.

A COMPRESS

A poultice is made from a crushed plant and is applied directly to the affected areas. Boil crushed plant parts for a few minutes to make a pulp, or mix powdered herbs with boiling water. Poultices are particularly useful for conditions such as bruises, wounds, and abscesses, helping to soothe and to draw out impurities.

Compresses are normally made by soaking a linen or muslin cloth in an infusion or decoction. The cloth is then placed on the affected area, where it can be held in place by a bandage or plastic wrap. Compresses can be hot or cold, and are generally milder than poultices.

OINTMENTS AND CREAMS

For external use, herbal ointments and creams are often prescribed. You can make your own by boiling the plant parts and adding a little pure oil (such as olive or sunflower), then simmering again until the water has been absorbed into the mixture. Stiffen the mixture with a little beeswax or cocoa butter to make a cream. The bain-marie method may also be useful. Creams and ointments should be kept in the refrigerator to maintain freshness and effectiveness.

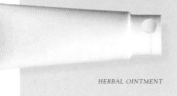

HERBAL OINTMENT

FLOWER ESSENCES

When buying flower essences you purchase a stock bottle of remedy – concentrated remedy from which personal remedies can be made. Do not use this undiluted. A personal remedy may contain up to six concentrates. Decide on the concentrates needed, put four drops of each into a clean 1 floz/30ml bottle, and add water and a teaspoon of brandy to act as a preservative. Shake well and label. Consult a practitioner for detailed instructions on making flower essences, and information on combinations and the conditions they treat.

FLOWER ESSENCE

ESSENTIAL OILS

Often used in therapies such as aromatherapy, the essential oils of a plant are those which contain its most active components. These oils can be extracted by steam distillation, but it is easier to buy essential oils in the shops. Essential oils are useful for making tinctures and ointments.

DILUTION

Many herbal oils can be applied neat to an external complaint. Others need to be diluted with oils (in the case of essential oils), water (in the case of some tinctures), or other fluids or creams.

ROSE CREAM

Other forms of treatment

THERE ARE MANY forms of gentle treatments which can be safely administered in the home. You can make your own flower essence by placing flowers in a glass bowl of spring water and leaving in strong sunlight for several hours, allowing the plant to energize the water.

INHALATION

Steam inhalation using drops of essential oils.

DIFFUSERS AND VAPORIZERS

These release the scent of essential oils or herbs into the air, providing natural fragrance while distributing their therapeutic benefits. Diffusers can be electrical, burners that use candles, or a simple ceramic ring that is warmed by a light bulb.

AROMATHERAPY

VAPORIZER

MASSAGE

The combination of touch and the therapeutic benefits of essential oils improves circulation, and releases tense muscles. Massage also ensures that the oils or herbal preparations are rubbed deep into the skin where they can enter the bloodstream.

MASSAGE

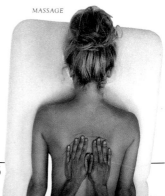

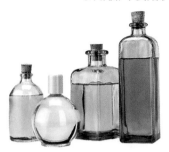

HERBAL PREPARATIONS IN OIL

BATHS

Herbs, plants, foodstuffs, and oils can be added to the bath for a whole body treatment, or to footbaths or facebaths.

INTERNAL USE

Some remedies can be taken internally. Speak to a practitioner if you are in doubt. As a rule of thumb, most essential oils should not be taken internally. Many herbs can be toxic in large amounts.

CAUTION

Never take anything internally that is meant for external use only.

REMEDIES KEY

These treatment symbols are used on the following pages.

Bath   Compress   Cream or lotion

Use damp cotton wool   Eat   Drink

Eyewash   Footbath   Inhale

Gargle   Massage   Mouthwash

Use neat   Paste   Poultice

Shampoo   Shower   Syrup

Use on a toothbrush   Vaporizer   Other treatment

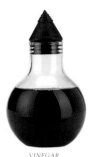

Vinegar

ACETIC ACID

VINEGAR IS OFTEN *used to preserve herbs. It also has many medicinal uses, and can be taken internally or applied externally. It can even be used in the bath – useful for soothing skin problems and easing thrush.*

VINEGAR

HOME REMEDIES

Properties and uses

• Vinegar is antiseptic and astringent, and excellent for urinary tract infections.

• Antifungal, used in the treatment of thrush.

• Apple cider is a good tonic, and can relieve a sore throat.

Vinegar can be drunk (warm with a little honey) to treat digestive disorders and urinary infections.

Apply vinegar to wasp stings to reduce swelling and ease discomfort.

Coughs, colds, and infections will respond to a cup of warm water with two tablespoons of vinegar and some honey. Arthritis and asthma may also be treated with the same drink, adding slightly more vinegar.

Apply cider vinegar to treat athlete's foot, ringworm, and eczema.

Drink vinegar daily to treat thrush, and apply (mixed with a little warm water) to the exterior of the vagina to ease itching.

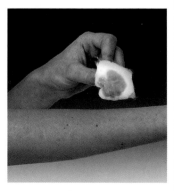

ABOVE *Use cotton wool to apply vinegar to a wasp sting.*

Onion

ALLIUM CEPA

THE BULB of the onion is used in cooking and medicinally. Like garlic and onion, it warms the body and stimulates the circulation. Onions have long been considered the mainstay of every household remedy chest.

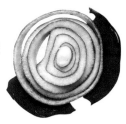

ONION

Properties and uses

- Onion causes "weeping" which releases toxins.
- Increases circulation and can relax muscles.
- Expectorant, antibacterial, and diuretic.
- Helps to reduce serum cholesterol after a fatty meal.
- May provide some protection against cancer.

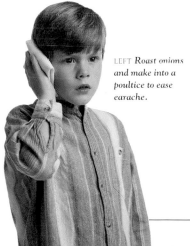

LEFT *Roast onions and make into a poultice to ease earache.*

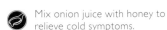 Mix onion juice with honey to relieve cold symptoms.

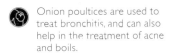 Onion poultices are used to treat bronchitis, and can also help in the treatment of acne and boils.

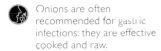 Onions are often recommended for gastric infections: they are effective cooked and raw.

Use a poultice of roasted onion for earaches

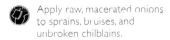 Apply raw, macerated onions to sprains, bruises, and unbroken chilblains.

Eat daily if you have a predisposition to heart disease or circulatory disorders.

HOME REMEDIES

GARLIC

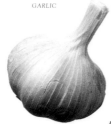

Garlic

ALLIUM SATIVUM

GARLIC CLOVE

GARLIC BELONGS *to the onion family, and is one of the best-known and most-used medicinal herbs. It has a strong odor, but its health-giving and preventative properties make this well worth enduring.*

Properties and uses

- Garlic is an antiseptic with antibiotic and antifungal actions.
- Antioxidant, decongestant.
- May help to reduce high blood-pressure.
- May prevent some cancers; in particular, stomach cancer.
- Treats infections of the stomach and respiratory system.
- Prevents heart disease and reduces the risk of atherosclerosis.

GARLIC SYRUP

Place 6 to 8 cloves of chopped, fresh garlic in a jar, and cover with 8 tablespoons of honey. Let stand for several days, and then strain. The garlic-infused honey can be given by the teaspoonful (one for children, four for adults), to boost the immune system and treat infections.

GARLIC SYRUP

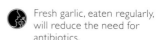 Fresh garlic, eaten regularly, will reduce the need for antibiotics.

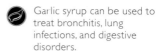 Garlic syrup can be used to treat bronchitis, lung infections, and digestive disorders.

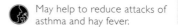 May help to reduce attacks of asthma and hay fever.

Infused oil can be used as a chest rub for respiratory or digestive ailments, or in the ear to reduce inflammation.

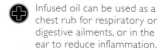 Fresh garlic juice is antifungal, and can be applied neat to fungal infections such as athlete's foot.

Chew roasted garlic cloves to improve the circulation.

The intestinal tract can be cleansed by adding mashed, raw garlic cloves to salads.

Celery

APIUM GRAVEOLENS

CELERY *CELERY SEEDS*

HIPPOCRATES, *the father of medicine, wrote that celery could be used to calm the nerves – its very high calcium level probably accounts for this recommendation. The seeds, leaves and edible root of the plant are used.*

Properties and uses

• Reduces high blood-pressure.
• A digestive, reduces spasm in the muscle of the intestinal tract and acts as an anti-inflammatory.
• May help in the treatment of arthritis and rheumatic disorders. In Japan, rheumatic patients are sometimes put on a celery-only diet.
• Seeds are anti-inflammatory.
• Stimulates the thyroid and pituitary glands.
• Possibly antioxidant.
• Helps clear uric acid from painful joints.
• Acts on the kidneys and is a mild diuretic.

CAUTION

Because celery may cause the uterus to contract, it should not be eaten during pregnancy.

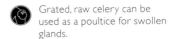
Grated, raw celery can be used as a poultice for swollen glands.

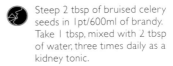
Steep 2 tbsp of bruised celery seeds in 1pt/600ml of brandy. Take 1 tbsp, mixed with 2 tbsp of water, three times daily as a kidney tonic.

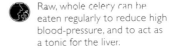
Raw, whole celery can be eaten regularly to reduce high blood-pressure, and to act as a tonic for the liver.

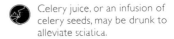
Celery juice, or an infusion of celery seeds, may be drunk to alleviate sciatica.

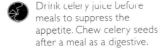
Drink celery juice before meals to suppress the appetite. Chew celery seeds after a meal as a digestive.

Celery root is said to be an aphrodisiac.

CELERY JUICE

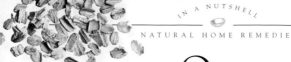

OATS

Oats

AVENA SATIVUM

THE OAT IS *a cereal plant, and is both extremely nutritious and useful therapeutically. Oats are one of the best sources of inositol, which is important for maintaining blood cholesterol levels. Eaten daily, they provide a wealth of excellent effects.*

Properties and uses
• Extremely rich in B vitamins and minerals.
• Antidepressant, and can be used to treat depression, stress, and nervous disorders. Often used in the treatment of addictions.
• A tonic for general debility, and used in the treatment of anorexia, and for convalescence and fatigue.
• Lowers blood cholesterol levels.
• Helps to control hormonal activity.
• Cleansing – internally and externally. May protect against bowel cancer when taken internally.
• Treatment of eczema.

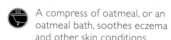
A compress of oatmeal, or an oatmeal bath, soothes eczema and other skin conditions.

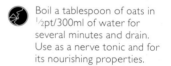
Boil a tablespoon of oats in 1/2pt/300ml of water for several minutes and drain. Use as a nerve tonic and for its nourishing properties.

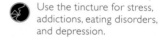
Use the tincture for stress, addictions, eating disorders, and depression.

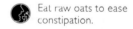
Eat raw oats to ease constipation.

Eating cooked oats will relieve fatigue.

HOME REMEDIES

RIGHT *Eating porridge daily for breakfast ensures a good oat intake.*

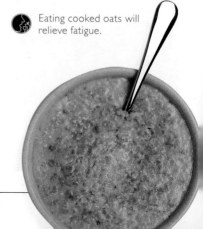

Cabbage

BRASSICA OLERACEA

CABBAGE HAS *traditionally been used for medicinal purposes as well as a food. It contains chemicals that may prevent cancer. The ancient Greeks used fresh white cabbage juice to relieve sore or infected eyes.*

CABBAGE

Properties and uses
- Reduces the pain of headaches and rheumatic disorders.
- An excellent anti-inflammatory.
- Soothes eczema and other itching or weeping skin conditions.
- May prevent cancer.
- Draws out infection.
- Red cabbage leaves form the basis of a good cough syrup.

 Make cabbage a regular part of your diet to help reduce the risk of cancer.

 A cabbage poultice can be applied to boils and infected cuts to draw out the infection.

 Applied to bruises and swelling, macerated cabbage leaves will encourage healing.

 Dab white cabbage juice on mouth ulcers, and use it to gargle if you have a sore throat.

 A warm cabbage compress, placed on the affected area, will reduce headaches and some neuralgias.

 Drink fresh cabbage juice to reduce the discomfort of gastric ulcers and bronchial infections. A cabbage leaf, lightly pounded, can be placed directly on the breast to relieve mastitis.

HOME REMEDIES

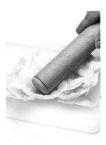

LEFT **Preparing a cabbage poultice.**

Marigold

MARIGOLD

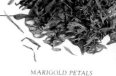

MARIGOLD PETALS

CALENDULA OFFICINALIS

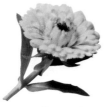

THIS POPULAR *garden plant has exceptional healing powers, and is used in many therapeutic disciplines such as homeopathy. For medicinal purposes, it is commonly known as "calendula."*

Properties and uses

- Uplifting.
- It is antiseptic and promotes quick healing of wounds.
- Relaxing.
- Healing – used internally and externally.
- Anti-inflammatory.
- Useful in the treatment of skin and eye disorders.
- A wonderful healing remedy for cuts and wounds.
- According to ancient diviners, calendula encourages prophetic dreams and makes them come true.

Calendula is also an important homeopathic remedy, which encourages the healing of wounds. Take it three times each day until the wound begins to heal, and clean it with a homeopathic "mother tincture," diluted in water.

 Apply tea or tincture as a compress for boils, spots, inflamed wounds, inflamed and painful varicose veins, and sore eyes.

 Drink a mild infusion for colic and abdominal cramping.

 Use as a mouthwash and gargle for sore throats, tonsillitis, chronic ear infections, mouth sores, and ulcers.

 Apply calendula lotion or cream to itchy skin rashes, grazes, cuts, eczema, and fungal infections.

 Smooth calendula ointment or infused oil on sore or chapped hands and lips.

CHAMOMILE FLOWER

Chamomile

CHAMOMILLA RECUTITA

CHAMOMILE *is probably the most versatile of all herbs, used medicinally for more than a thousand years. Its healing properties are excellent for skin conditions, including eczema. It is used to reduce fever, particularly in children.*

Properties and uses
• Anti-parasitic and antiseptic, used internally and externally.
• Digestive – reduces most digestive upsets.
• Anti-inflammatory, particularly for skin conditions.
• Reduces spasm.
• A valuable homeopathic remedy, particularly for intolerable neuralgic pain, toothache, joint and muscle pain, colic, heavy periods, and during labor. Chamomile essential oil is ideal for massage, to relax and restore, and will help to treat even the most chronic insomnia.

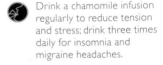 Drink a chamomile infusion regularly to reduce tension and stress; drink three times daily for insomnia and migraine headaches.

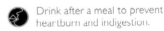 Drink after a meal to prevent heartburn and indigestion.

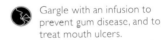 Gargle with an infusion to prevent gum disease, and to treat mouth ulcers.

Use an infusion as an eyewash to treat conjunctivitis, and strained eyes.

Chamomile tea can ease teething and digestive problems in children.

Rinsing fair hair with chamomile will bring out natural highlights.

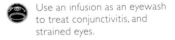 Add a handful of herbs to the bath to relax and restore.

 CHAMOMILE

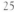

Lemon

CITRUS LIMON

LEMON LEAVES

LEMON

LEMONS ARE *rich in vitamin C, and have a cleansing effect on the digestive system. They have a wide range of therapeutic properties. The leaves or the whole fruit may be used according to requirements.*

Properties and uses

• Improves the body's ability to expel toxins. Useful for skin problems such as acne and boils.

• One of the most powerful natural astringents: use on cuts and grazes to stop bleeding.

• Antibacterial and antiviral properties; excellent for halting the progression of infections.

• Controls bladder and kidney infections.

LEMON DRINK

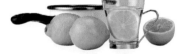

HOME REMEDIES

Lemon strengthens the immune system and helps relieve the symptoms of colds and flu. It can also be beneficial in the treatment of other infections. Infuse three or four sliced lemons in 1pt/600ml of water, and boil, uncovered, until liquid is reduced by half. Add a little honey to sweeten.

Use pure lemon juice on wasp stings to relieve the pain.

May be useful in the treatment of hemorrhoids, kidney stones, gallstones, and varicose veins.

Put a few drops of undiluted lemon juice on cold sores, and repeat several times a day.

A drop of lemon juice will benefit ulcers on the tongue and in the mouth.

ESSENTIAL OIL

Lemon essential oil is a very good tonic for the circulatory system, and improves capillary health. It has a purifying effect and can be used for infections of every type – parasitic, bacterial, fungal, and viral. It is good for respiratory infections, and can be put in a vaporizer to treat colds and flu.

Grapefruit

CITRUS PARADISI

GRAPEFRUIT
SEGMENT

LIKE ALL *citrus fruit, grapefruit is rich in vitamin C and potassium. It is an excellent cleanser for the digestive and urinary systems, and the peel has many therapeutic properties. Grapefruit essential oil is popular in aromatherapy.*

Properties and uses

- Cleanses the digestive and urinary systems. It is often recommended by naturopaths.
- Strengthens the respiratory system, and aids respiration.
- Invigorating – used as a tonic.
- Relieves symptoms of colds and flu.
- May help in the treatment of osteoarthritis.
- Balances the nervous system.

ESSENTIAL OIL

Grapefruit essential oil is excellent for liverish complaints, headaches, constipation, and hangovers. It can help to strengthen immunity against colds.

GRAPEFRUIT

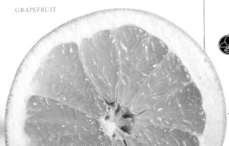

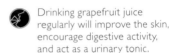 Drinking grapefruit juice regularly will improve the skin, encourage digestive activity, and act as a urinary tonic.

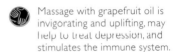 Massage with grapefruit oil is invigorating and uplifting, may help to treat depression, and stimulates the immune system.

Local massage with a few drops of essential oil in a carrier oil will relieve headaches.

Drinking grapefruit juice with iron supplements, or foods rich in iron, increases the absorption of iron in the body.

Detoxifies the liver, and can ease chronic liver conditions. May help to reduce the severity of a hangover.

Used in steam inhalation or burnt in a room, grapefruit oil is good for treating colds, flu, and respiratory problems.

HOME REMEDIES

CUCUMBER SEEDS

Cucumber

CUCUMIS SATIVIS

CUCUMBER IS *a popular vegetable, widely used in folk medicine to reduce heat and inflammation. It is a rich source of vitamin C, and can be used externally to cool and cleanse.*

CUCUMBER

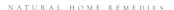

Properties and uses

- Diuretic.
- Cleansing, particularly for skin disorders.
- Used in the treatment of gout and arthritis.
- Anti-inflammatory – soothes inflamed skin.
- May help to treat lung and chest disorders.
- Drink cucumber juice to treat inflammatory conditions, such as arthritis.

CUCUMBER SLICES

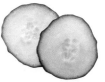

LEFT *To soothe the eyes, lie down for half an hour with a slice of cucumber on each eye.*

H O M E   R E M E D I E S

Place a cucumber slice over strained or inflamed eyes to reduce swelling and soothe.

Cool sunburn by applying fresh cucumber or cucumber juice.

Ground dried cucumber seeds are used to treat tapeworm.

Cucumber juice, drunk daily, may help to control eczema, arthritis, and gout. It is a mild diuretic.

Skin conditions respond to cucumber. Eat the whole cucumber.

Cucumber juice acts as a kidney tonic.

Use cucumber ointment externally on inflammatory skin conditions.

EUCALYPTUS

Eucalyptus

EUCALYPTUS GLOBULUS; EUCALYPTUS CITRIODORA

THE EUCALYPTUS *tree is also known as the gum tree, and its leaves and older branches are used to produce one of the most important essential oils available.*

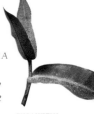

EUCALYPTUS
LEAVES

Properties and uses

• A strong antibiotic, which encourages the action of the immune system.

• Very good expectorant, particularly for deep-seated colds that have settled on the chest.

• Anti-rheumatic, for many musculo-skeletal conditions, ranging from general aches and pains to arthritis.

• Excellent for gastric infections, particularly when combined with fennel.

• Lowers body temperature, and is used to reduce fevers.

• Disinfectant.

Inhale eucalyptus essential oil to treat pneumonia, bronchitis, asthma, colds, and flu – it opens the breathing tubes and eases congestion.

Use one or two drops in massage for rheumatic conditions.

Dilute and use externally for skin infections: antibiotic properties prevent and treat infection.

Dab neat on stings and insect bites to ease itching.

Place a few drops of oil in a footbath to treat athlete's foot.

Add one drop of oil to your shampoo to rid hair of nits. Use regularly to prevent reinfestation.

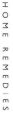

HOME REMEDIES

CAUTION

Use cautiously when pregnant, or when treating babies. Effective in small doses.

RIGHT *A few drops of eucalyptus oil in a footbath can be used to treat athlete's foot.*

Cloves

CLOVES

EUGENICA CARYOPHYLLATA

CLOVES ARE *the fruit of an aromatic herb, and have a variety of culinary and medicinal uses. Buy dried cloves from the supermarket, and oil of cloves from the pharmacy.*

ABOVE *Oil of cloves may be rubbed on the gums to relieve toothache.*

Properties and uses

• Antiseptic and analgesic – use for treating toothache.

• Warming, and therefore valuable to people prone to colds.

• Calms the digestive system.

• Anti-inflammatory, when used locally on swellings.

• Eliminates parasites from the body.

CAUTION

Cloves can cause uterine contractions, and should not be used in any form during pregnancy.

BELOW *Inhale an infusion of cloves to clear the lungs and refresh.*

Oil of cloves can be placed directly on the gums.

Dab a tiny amount of neat oil on insect bites.

Clove tea is warming, and can encourage the body to sweat, which is helpful in cases of high fever or vomiting.

Oil of cloves may be used in a long labor to hasten birth.

Clove tea can be used to soothe wind and ease nausea – particularly travel sickness.

A clove and orange pomander can be used as an insect repellent in cupboards.

Steep cloves in boiling water and then simmer. Strain and use the remaining liquid as a mild sedative.

HOME REMEDIES

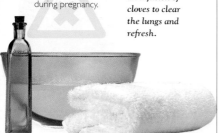

Fennel

FOENICULUM VULGARE

FENNEL IS AN *aromatic herb with culinary, cosmetic, and medicinal uses. The seeds, roots, and leaves are eaten for their digestive and diuretic properties.*

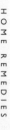

FENNEL

Properties and uses

• Fennel is beneficial for ailments of the digestive and respiratory systems, particularly for coughs and colds, intestinal gas, and colic.
• Fennel helps to expel gas from the gut.
• A gentle laxative.
• Mild expectorant.
• Helps to produce milk in nursing mothers.
• Anti-inflammatory – often used in eye conditions.
• Essential oil of fennel is a gentle, warming oil used for digestive disorders, and to promote the flow of milk in nursing mothers. Some therapists use the oil as an antidepressant.

 A tea made with fennel seeds will ease indigestion, and reduce flatulence.

 Fennel syrup can be used to treat coughs, shortness of breath, and wheezing.

 Fennel – fresh and dried – improves liver function.

 Fresh fennel is a diuretic, and helps to cleanse the liver, spleen, gallbladder, and blood. Eat regularly in salads, soups, and breads.

 Fennel tea may be used as a gargle.

 Fennel oil, mixed with honey, can be taken for coughs.

 Boil the seeds to make an eyewash for conjunctivitis and sore, inflamed eyes.

FENNEL
GARNISH

CAUTION

Do not use fennel oil if you are pregnant.

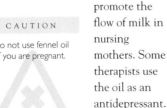

Licorice

GLYCYRRHIZA GLABRA

LICORICE ROOT

LICORICE IS *a pretty, blue-flowered perennial, grown mainly in Europe. The sweet substance is obtained mainly from the roots, and is used medicinally and as a flavoring. The root is said to increase sexual vitality.*

Properties and uses

- Expectorant and anti-inflammatory, making it excellent for stubborn coughs and lung infections.
- Mild laxative.
- Adrenal tonic.
- Detoxifies the body; in the Far East licorice is used to rid the body of poisons such as salmonella, or drugs.
- Raises blood-pressure, and can be used in the treatment of low blood-pressure.
- Inhibits gastric secretions, making it useful for treatment of gastric ulcers.
- Stimulates the kidneys and bowels.

A strong infusion can protect against and heal ulcers. Take three times daily.

Steep licorice root with a blend of other soothing herb teas to treat gastric disorders, and to stimulate kidneys and bowel.

Licorice syrup can be used to treat persistent coughs, and to reduce the incidence of asthma attacks.

Used with other strengthening herbs, such as ginseng, for exhaustion.

Use creams or pastes for inflamed psoriasis, and hot and weeping skin conditions.

CAUTION

Large doses can cause water retention and exacerbate high blood-pressure. Avoid in pregnancy.

LICORICE LEAF

Witch hazel

HAMAMELIS VIRGINIANA

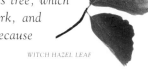

WITCH HAZEL *is a common deciduous tree, which originated in America. Its leaves, bark, and roots are used for medicinal purposes because of their anti-inflammatory properties.*

WITCH HAZEL LEAF

Properties and uses

- Soothes swellings and reduces inflammation and bleeding.
- Will encourage healing of bruises, sprains and bleeding hemorrhoids.
- Antiseptic – can be used as a facial wash, and diluted to wash cuts and grazes.

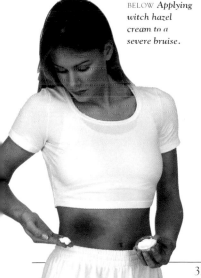

BELOW **Applying witch hazel cream to a severe bruise.**

Apply externally (as a decoction, tincture or cream) for bruising, and hemorrhoids or varicose veins.

Use as a compress for sprains and strains.

Dilute one part witch hazel to 20 parts boiled, cooled water, and use as an eyewash for sore and inflamed eyes.

Add to the bath to reduce aches and pains of rheumatic conditions.

HOMEOPATHY

The main action of the homeopathic remedy Hamamelis (witch hazel) is on the veins and arteries – i.e., hemorrhoids, nosebleeds, varicose veins, and hemorrhages.

HOME REMEDIES

BARLEY

Barley

HORDEUM SATIVUM VULGARE

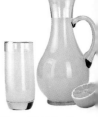

LEMON BARLEY

BARLEY IS RICH *in minerals (calcium and potassium) and B-complex vitamins, which makes it beneficial for convalescents. Barley has been used for its restorative qualities for thousands of years.*

Properties and uses
- Nutritious.
- Anti-inflammatory – particularly for the urinary and digestive systems.
- Used in the treatment of respiratory disorders.
- Taken daily, it may lower cholesterol levels.

BARLEY WATER

Add 2 tablespoons of pearl barley to 1pt/600ml of water and boil for 10 minutes. Strain, and add the barley to a fresh 1pt/600ml of water. Boil for another 10 minutes. Strain out the barley and serve the water warm or cold, with lemon and honey.

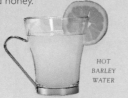

HOT BARLEY WATER

Barley water eases dry, tickling coughs.

Barley water can be used for urinary tract infections and cystitis, and can ease flatulence and colic.

Cooked barley is easily digested and nutritious, and is a traditional remedy for constipation and diarrhea.

Barley water reduces acid in the spleen if drunk twice a day for a month.

Make a poultice of barley flour to reduce inflammation of the skin.

Barley may help to prevent heart disease, as it stabilizes blood-pressure.

Eat in soups and stews when convalescing.

HOME REMEDIES

Yogurt

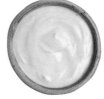

YOGURT

As a food, *yogurt is a rich source of protein, and all the vitamins and minerals normally found in milk. Live yogurt, which contains active bacteria, should be eaten to increase the healthy bacteria in the body, which help it to fight infection.*

Properties and uses

• Live yogurt is antifungal, and can be used in the treatment of thrush.

• Live yogurt may help to reduce blood cholesterol levels.

BELOW *Use natural yogurt as a cleanser: apply with a pad of cotton wool.*

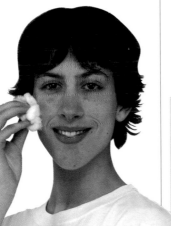

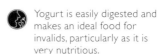 Yogurt is easily digested and makes an ideal food for invalids, particularly as it is very nutritious.

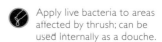 Apply live bacteria to areas affected by thrush; can be used internally as a douche.

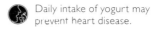 Daily intake of yogurt may prevent heart disease.

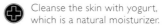 Cleanse the skin with yogurt, which is a natural moisturizer.

HOME REMEDIES

ANTIBIOTICS

We take antibiotics to kill infections, but unfortunately they kill beneficial bacteria at the same time. To renew the flora in the intestines, eat live yogurt daily for a few weeks.

Lavender

LAVANDULA VERA, L. OFFICINALIS

LAVENDER IS ONE *of the most versatile of all herbs, with a long history of medicinal and cosmetic use. The whole plant is aromatic, and can be used for treatment, but the flowers alone are distilled to make the essential oil.*

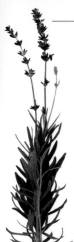

LAVENDER

HOME REMEDIES

Properties and uses

• Antiseptic, and may reduce severity of urinary tract infections, as well as encouraging healing.

• Anti-spasmodic – may help treat asthma and coughs.

• Antiseptic qualities make it excellent for treating flu, colds and other viral infections.

• Intestinal stimulant, which reduces colic and stomach disorders; may reduce diarrhea, nausea and indigestion.

• Generates skin cells, and is useful for skin conditions such as eczema and psoriasis.

• Analgesic, and thus beneficial for headaches, migraines, and neurological pain.

• Helpful for high blood-pressure, regulates scanty periods. Helpful for general stress, palpitations, faintness, and dizziness.

Place lavender flowers in a muslin bag in the bath to soothe aches and pains.

A hot lavender compress reduces inflammation and eases pain locally.

Apply oil neat to bruises, minor burns, bites and stings for instant relief.

A few drops on the temple will ease a headache.

Use the essential oil to relieve the pain of neuralgia and rheumatic disorders.

Put a few drops of lavender oil on a handkerchief by the bed, or your child's cot, to soothe and encourage sleep. Lavender is excellent for children's ailments such as sleep disorders, nappy rash (in an ointment or cream: add a few drops to zinc oxide cream to provide barrier protection).

Apple
MALUS SPECIES

APPLE

THE APPLE *has many uses in traditional medicine, and the old adage "To eat an apple going to bed, will make the doctor beg his bread" has been justified by research showing that apples are excellent detoxifiers, and that apple juice can destroy viruses.*

Properties and uses
- Cleans teeth and strengthens gums.
- Lowers cholesterol levels.
- Antiviral action.
- Detoxifies.
- Protects from pollution binding to toxins in the body and carrying them out.
- Neutralizes indigestion.
- Prevents constipation.
- Soothing and antiseptic.

CAUTION

Apple seeds can be toxic when taken in large amounts.

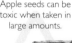

APPLE JUICE

Throughout history, apples have been considered symbols of life and immortality. In some places, where there is a belief in reincarnation, apples are buried as food for the dead.

 Eat raw apples regularly, as a detoxicant, for gout and rheumatism.

 To prevent viruses from settling in, and to reduce their duration, eat an apple (or drink a glass of apple juice) three times a day.

 Peeled, grated apples can be used as a poultice for sprains.

 For indigestion, heartburn, and other digestive disorders, eat an apple with meals.

 Two apples a day can reduce cholesterol levels.

 As a treatment for intestinal infections, hoarseness, rheumatism, and fatigue, increase your daily intake of apples to up to 2lb/1kg.

Grated apple, mixed with live yogurt, may be helpful in cases of diarrhea.

H O M E R E M E D I E S

Honey

FOR CENTURIES *honey has been used as an antiseptic, for external and internal conditions, and as a tonic for overall good health. Each country has a distinctive type of honey.*

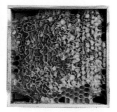

HONEYCOMB

Properties and uses

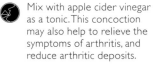

HONEY BEE

- Sedative.
- Nourishing.
- Antibacterial, for external and internal infections. There are active antibiotic properties in unpasteurized honey.
- For hay fever, eat a little of the local honey to encourage your body to build up an immunity to indigenous pollen.
- Apply a honey compress to cuts and bruises.
- Smear set honey on ringworm several times a day. Leave uncovered.

BELOW **Honey and lemon syrup is a pleasant-tasting cough medicine.**

Mix with apple cider vinegar as a tonic. This concoction may also help to relieve the symptoms of arthritis, and reduce arthritic deposits.

Honey ointment can soothe and encourage healing of sores in the mouth or vagina.

Honey water can be used as an eye lotion (particularly good for conjunctivitis and other infectious conditions).

Gargle with honey water to soothe a sore throat and ease respiratory problems.

Honey and lemon drink is a traditional cough remedy.

Honey is an excellent moisturizer, and can be used as a revitalizing face mask.

Honey warmed with a little milk can be used as a sedative.

HOME REMEDIES

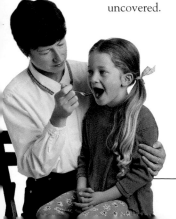

Peppermint

MENTHA PIPERITA

PEPPERMINT

PEPPERMINT IS *a cooling herb, and it will help to cool and detoxify the body – particularly the liver. The leaves of this plant are used medicinally and for cooking.*

Properties and uses

• Treats food poisoning, diarrhea, colic and gastric flu.

• Refreshing, acts as a general tonic, helps to treat migraine.

• Expectorant, decongestant, and anti-spasmodic properties are useful for treating asthma, bronchitis, sinusitis, and colds and coughs.

• Peppermint eases nausea.

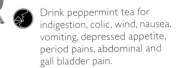
Drink peppermint tea for indigestion, colic, wind, nausea, vomiting, depressed appetite, period pains, abdominal and gall bladder pain.

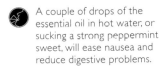
A couple of drops of the essential oil in hot water, or sucking a strong peppermint sweet, will ease nausea and reduce digestive problems.

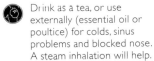
Drink as a tea, or use externally (essential oil or poultice) for colds, sinus problems and blocked nose. A steam inhalation will help.

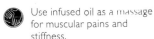
Use infused oil as a massage for muscular pains and stiffness.

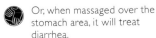
Or, when massaged over the stomach area, it will treat diarrhea.

Good as a mouthwash and as a footbath for aching feet.

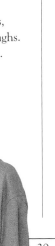
RIGHT
Drinking peppermint tea.

HOME REMEDIES

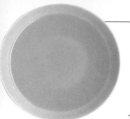

Olive

OLEA EUROPEA

ABOVE **Olive oil:
essential to
Mediterranean cuisine.**

THE EVERGREEN *olive tree is native to the
Mediterranean. Its leaves and the oil of its fruit are
used both in cooking and medicinally.*

Properties and uses

- Olive oil is rich in vitamin E, and is believed to help lower cholesterol levels in the body.
- It may reduce the risk of circulatory disease and nervous disorders.
- Useful in the treatment of gastric disorders: reduces the secretion of gastric juices.
- Olive oil can be used to treat constipation.
- Soothes the itching of eczema, and moisturizes dry skin, hair, and scalp.

Rub olive oil into patches of eczema, dandruff, and psoriasis to reduce itching and encourage healing.

Olives and olive oil, as part of a daily diet, will reduce the risk of circulatory problems and will lower cholesterol. Scientists recommend that we buy olive oil from the first pressing of the olives, known as extra-virgin olive oil, as it has the highest concentration of beneficial ingredients.

Eat olives to ease constipation.

LEFT **Olives have a wide
range of medicinal uses,
as well as being a staple
cooking ingredient.**

OLIVE FLOWER ESSENCE

For those who are exhausted due to overwork or over-exertion; people who have no energy or strength left and for whom life is no longer fun. The remedy revives and replaces lost energy. Also good for when someone is being mentally stretched, or after illness.

HOME REMEDIES

Bread

BREAD – *particularly wholegrain bread – is an excellent source of carbohydrate and B-complex vitamins. These vitamins maintain the health of the nervous system and ensure healthy functioning of body systems.*

Properties and uses
- Nutritious.
- Anti-inflammatory.
- Styptic (stops bleeding).

HOME REMEDIES

TRADITIONAL USE

Traditionally, bread was used as a poultice, and applied as a styptic to stop the bleeding of wounds.

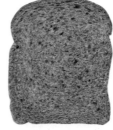

ABOVE **Wholemeal bread supplies dietary fiber, which is vital for intestinal health.**

TO MAKE A POULTICE

Remove crusts and chop bread into small cubes. Put into a pan with a little water or milk, and simmer for a few minutes.

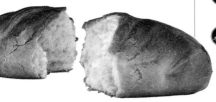

BELOW **Bread is an important part of a nutritious diet.**

 Apply cold bread to closed eyes to reduce the inflammation of conjunctivitis, and soothe itching.

 Apply a warm bread poultice to infected cuts to reduce itching and pain.

 Apply fresh bread to shallow wounds, to help stop bleeding.

 Help to bring out a boil, and ease the pain of it, by applying a hot bread poultice.

Avocado

PERSICA AMERICANA GRATISSIMA

AVOCADO

AVOCADOS ARE *rich in vitamins A, C and E, some B-complex vitamins, and potassium. Because they contain some protein and starch, and are a good source of mono-unsaturated fats, they are considered to be a complete food.*

Properties and uses
- Excellent restorative food, particularly for convalescents.
- Traditionally used for sexual problems.
- For skin disorders.
- Antioxidant.
- Used to treat circulatory problems.
- Digestive.
- Antibacterial and antifungal.

LEFT **An avocado face mask helps treat skin problems.**

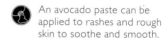 An avocado paste can be applied to rashes and rough skin to soothe and smooth.

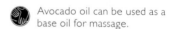 Avocado oil can be used as a base oil for massage.

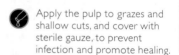 Apply the pulp to grazes and shallow cuts, and cover with sterile gauze, to prevent infection and promote healing.

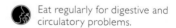 Eat regularly for digestive and circulatory problems.

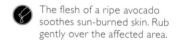 The flesh of a ripe avocado soothes sun-burned skin. Rub gently over the affected area.

Make a face mask for the skin by mashing a ripe avocado with a little olive oil. Smooth over the face and affected area (e.g. patches of mild eczema) and rinse off after 15 minutes.

HOME REMEDIES

Rosemary

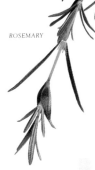

ROSEMARY

ROSMARINUS OFFICINALIS

ROSEMARY IS *a popular herb, and the rosemary bush grows easily in most soils. The plant is characterized by its needle-like leaves, aromatic scent and attractive blue flowers.*

Properties and uses

- Rosemary is refreshing and improves circulation.
- Stimulates and nourishes the nervous system, making it a good, gentle tonic.
- Encourages the digestion of foods – particularly fatty foods such as lamb.
- Rinsing your hair in an infusion of rosemary adds shine.

CAUTION

Avoid rosemary if you suffer from high blood-pressure.

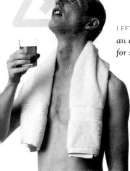

LEFT **Rosemary is an excellent gargle for sore throats.**

 Drink an infusion, eat fresh, or add to the bath, for circulatory conditions.

 As tea or tincture for depression and headaches associated with gastric upsets.

 Eat regularly for poor digestion or gall bladder disorders.

 Gargle an infusion for sore throats; useful substitute for sage during pregnancy.

 Rosemary vinegar keeps hair in good condition and reduces dandruff. Use 2 tbs/30ml in the rinsing water when you wash your hair.

 Inhale to unblock sinuses.

 Massage oil into the abdomen for digestive spasms and into cellulite.

HOME REMEDIES

Sage

SALVIA OFFICINALIS

SAGE LEAF

RED SAGE

RED SAGE *is normally used for healing purposes, although the properties of regular garden (green) sage are very similar. Grow sage in a sunny spot.*

Properties and uses

- Anti-inflammatory.
- Can reduce hot flushes in the menopause.
- Strengthens the lungs: used to treat respiratory problems including asthma.
- Carminative, and used to treat digestive disorders.
- Tonic for nervous disorders.
- Strong tea or tincture as a gargle and mouthwash for sore throats, laryngitis, mouth ulcers, and inflamed gums.

CAUTION

Do not take in therapeutic doses in pregnancy, with epilepsy or with high blood-pressure. Avoid when breastfeeding.

Drink as a tea for hot flushes and to dry up breast milk.

Drink as a tea or tincture for nervous disorders – including depression and conditions such as ME – as well as for indigestion and other digestive disorders.

Drink cold tea or tincture for night sweats.

Use an infusion for greasy and spotty skin.

An infusion may restore color to gray hair.

Drink one cup regularly as a tonic – particularly useful for women and the elderly.

Sage essential oil is warming, and can be used in massage for rheumatic disorders and after a cold.

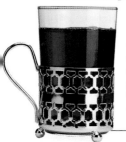

LEFT **A cup of sage tea, drunk regularly, makes a useful tonic, particularly for women and the elderly.**

HOME REMEDIES

Elderflower

SAMBUCUS NIGRA

THE FLOWERS, *leaves and berries of the elderflower plant are used for herbal remedies. Homeopaths use Sambucus nigra both to treat conditions accompanied by profuse perspiration, and for severe coughs.*

ELDERFLOWER

Properties and uses

• Drying and restorative for nose lining, eyes, and sinuses.

• Diuretic.

• Used to treat coughs, colic, diarrhea, sore throats, asthma, and flu.

• Kidney and lung tonic.

• Helps to strengthen the chest against infection.

• Elderberries are laxative.

• Ointment sooths nappy rash and other skin problems.

• Children can drink a mild infusion (sweetened with a little honey) to ease colds and encourage normal breathing.

• Elder leaf ointment works well on itchy and painful piles.

• Elderberry wine is a traditional drink for neuralgia and sciatica.

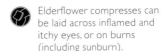
Elderflower compresses can be laid across inflamed and itchy eyes, or on burns (including sunburn).

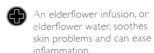
An elderflower infusion, or elderflower water, soothes skin problems and can ease inflammation.

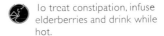
To treat constipation, infuse elderberries and drink while hot.

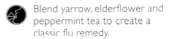
Blend yarrow, elderflower and peppermint tea to create a classic flu remedy.

Drink the tea, or take a few drops of the tincture in some warm water, three times daily, for respiratory disorders (particularly acute disorders such as colds and flu).

HOME REMEDIES

ELDERBERRIES

NATURAL HOME REMEDIES

Mustard

SINAPSIS ALBA, BRASSICA NIGRA

FOR MEDICINAL *purposes the leaves, flowers, seeds, and oils of the black mustard are used. Only the seeds of the white mustard are suitable.*

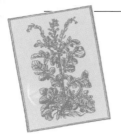

MUSTARD

Properties and uses

• Black mustard and white mustard are warming, and can be used to draw infection or congestion away from its source (for example, in the case of nasal congestion, or an abscess).

• Rubefacient qualities make it useful for respiratory and circulatory disorders.

• Mustard flour is an antiseptic and deodorizer.

• Mustard oil can be used for pain relief in arthritic conditions.

• An expectorant, and a powerful emetic.

A mustard footbath (1 tsp/5ml of mustard powder added to a bowl of hot water) is a traditional remedy for colds, circulatory problems, and headaches.

A mustard poultice can be applied to the chest to relieve infection and congestion.

Mustard essential oil can be used externally for neuralgia; gently massage a little oil on the affected area a few times a day.

A poultice of crushed seeds, or essential oil, can be applied to areas affected by rheumatism, sciatica, and lumbago.

LEFT **Mustard essential oil helps relieve neuralgia.**

CAUTION

Mustard seeds can burn the skin: use carefully. Avoid contact with mucous membranes, and with sensitive skin.

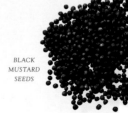

BLACK MUSTARD SEEDS

HOME REMEDIES

Bicarbonate of Soda

BAKING SODA

BAKING SODA is a powder traditionally used as a raising agent when baking. Baking soda is used in many natural remedies, and used on its own for its soothing and neutralizing properties.

RIGHT **Applying baking soda paste to a sting.**

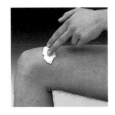

Properties and uses

• Anti-inflammatory, particularly for skin conditions.
• Natural bleach for teeth. Reduces the agents that cause bad breath.
• Alkaline, and so neutralizes acids.

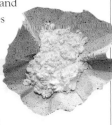

CAUTION

Do not take baking soda if you have high blood-pressure or heart trouble. Do not give to children.

ABOVE **Bicarbonate of soda is a white powder.**

 Drink 1 tsp/5ml of baking soda in water every hour for three hours, at the onset of cystitis.

 A paste of baking soda and water can be applied to nappy rash to reduce inflammation and irritation.

 Drink a solution of baking soda and hot water (1 tsp/5ml for every ⅓pt/225ml) to reduce flatulence and ease indigestion.

 For bee stings, extract the sting and apply a paste of baking soda and water to neutralize.

 The juice of half a lemon mixed with 1 tsp/5ml of baking soda and warm water will help ease a headache. Drink every 15 minutes until pain is reduced.

 Brush your teeth with baking soda, a natural whitener.

HOME REMEDIES

Dandelion

DANDELION FLOWERS

TARAXACUM OFFICINALIS

THE LEAVES, *flowers and roots of the common dandelion are a mainstay of herbal medicine, best known for their tonic and diuretic properties. The fresh leaves are a delicious addition to salads, and are very nourishing.*

Properties and uses

• An excellent diuretic and kidney tonic.

• Cleansing, by neutralizing the acids in the blood.

• Dandelion root coffee is an excellent liver tonic, and can be used to treat chronic and acute liver conditions.

• Dandelion root may be decocted and used to treat and prevent gallstones.

• Nourishing – the whole plant is rich in vitamins and minerals.

DANDELION LEAF

• Stimulates metabolism and cell respiration.

• Anti-inflammatory – often used in the treatment of arthritis, gout and mastitis.

• Stimulates the digestive system.

LEFT *The French word for dandelion, "pissenlit," refers to its diuretic qualities!*

Drink as a tea or coffee to treat water retention.

The fresh white sap of the stalks will eliminate warts when used regularly.

Drink as a tea to ease the discomfort of cystitis.

Dandelion tea or coffee can be drunk for most chronic and wasting diseases because it helps the body to cope with strong drugs.

Combine with poke root and marigold, and apply locally to treat mastitis.

Drink dandelion tea regularly to prevent PMS.

The leaves are infused for conditions such as arthritis and gout.

HOME REMEDIES

Nettle

URTICA DIOICA

NETTLE

NETTLE, *named Urtica, or Urtica urens for therapeutic purposes, is used for a wide variety of health conditions, and in cooking. The whole plant is rich in vitamins C and A, and iron, making it a good tonic.*

Properties and uses

- Nettle is diuretic and astringent.
- Will cleanse blood for anemia (detoxicant).
- Will soothe sore, blistered, swollen skin and rashes.
- Improves the metabolism and will help with weight problems.
- Improves function of the pancreas.
- Increases milk production in breastfeeding mothers.
- Can be used to treat urticaria, gout, urinary infections, rheumatism, and neuritis.

RIGHT **Drink nettle tea for urinary infections.**

 An infusion made from the fresh nettles will treat skin, hair, eyes, or arthritic joints.

 Drink nettle tea for urinary tract infections, cystitis, and to treat chilblains.

 Used internally and externally, nettles may give relief to sufferers of hay fever and other allergies, including skin allergies.

 A compress made by steeping a cloth in nettle tea will soothe burns.

 May reduce blood-pressure.

 Nettle acts as a tonic for the kidneys and liver, helping to rid the body of wastes and toxins.

 Drink regularly to increase resistance to allergic reactions, and to reduce severity of period problems.

Cranberry

VACCINIUM OXYCOCCUS VAR. PALUSTRIS

CRANBERRIES *are small, acidic berries, which are rich in vitamin C, and contain a substance which is excellent for fighting infection.*

CRANBERRIES

Properties and uses

- Has an antiseptic action on the urinary system.
- Used to control asthma.
- Improves the health of the circulatory system.
- Aids the treatment of kidney stones.

Cranberries contain a substance that affects the acidity of the urine and fights bacteria. A daily glass of cranberry juice will prevent and treat cystitis, and discourage kidney stones.

Crushed cranberries, boiled in distilled water, and skinned, can be added to a cup of warm water to overcome an asthma attack. The berries contain an active ingredient similar to the drugs used to control asthma.

HOME REMEDIES

BELOW **Cranberries are a weapon against the perennial complaint of cystitis.**

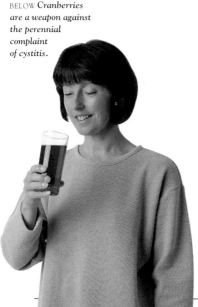

CRANBERRY SAUCE

Rich in vitamin C, cranberries don't deserve only to be eaten with the Christmas Turkey! Try serving cranberry sauce with yogurt or ice-cream. To make a sauce, cook the cranberries briefly in a syrup of water and a little sugar.

Ginger

ZINGIBER OFFICINALIS

GINGER IS A *plant with a spicy, warming aroma. The root of the plant is used in cooking and in medicine. It can be purchased fresh or dried.*

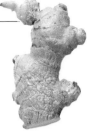

GINGER ROOT

Properties and uses

• Digestive aid – can stimulate the digestive process and tone the entire system.

• Detoxicant – cleanses the body, prevents colds, and soothes the respiratory system.

• Warming, slightly antiseptic, and promotes internal secretions.

• Eases nausea.

• Encourages circulation, and decreases muscular pains.

CAUTION

People suffering from gastric or peptic ulcers should avoid ginger.

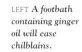

LEFT **A footbath containing ginger oil will ease chilblains.**

Ginger tea can ease nausea, and calm any internal spasms (for example, colic and IBS).

Powdered ginger, ginger tea and crystallized ginger will reduce morning sickness and ease travel sickness.

A poultice of fresh ginger may help to ease the discomfort of rheumatism.

Chewing fresh ginger can relieve toothache.

Used in massage, or inhaled, ginger can encourage the immune system and help to reduce the incidence of respiratory infections.

Use a few drops of oil or tincture in a foot or hand bath for chilblains and poor circulation.

A bath containing hot ginger tea will treat fevers, chest colds and flu.

HOME REMEDIES

Using home remedies

THE HOLISTIC APPROACH

Most home remedies are safe. Their use can save many a trip to the physician. If you are concerned about any health matter, it is best to see your physician or alternative practitioner before attempting to treat yourself at home. Home remedies are appropriate for most illnesses that are not life-threatening. They can normally be taken alongside orthodox medical care – although you must tell your physician about any remedies you are using yourself.

Many remedies work best if they are prescribed according to individual needs. If remedies don't seem to be having any effect, make an appointment to see a practitioner in the appropriate discipline – for example, a homeopath, a herbalist, or an aromatherapist.

TAKE CARE

Remember, natural medicine is not risk-free. Many herbs and plants can be toxic in large doses, and others should not be taken internally. Never take essential oils internally unless recommended to do so by a registered aromatherapist. Take doses that are appropriate for your age, your physical condition, and your ailment, and you should soon see results. Home remedies occasionally produce dramatic results; other times, as in the case of eczema, the course of treatment will take some time.

BELOW *Consult an alternative medicine practitioner if you have queries about remedies.*

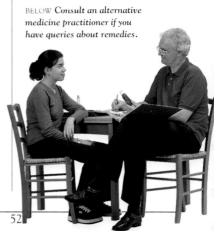

Common ailments

MANY COMMON *illnesses can be treated by natural home remedies instead of, or alongside, orthodox medicine. Always tell your physician about any treatments you are using, when you go for a consultation.*

ALLERGIES
• Eat the local honey if you suffer from hay fever.
• Honey and apple cider can be drunk in a glass of warm water to prevent allergies.
• Ginseng powder may prevent allergic attacks.
• Drink nettle tea to increase resistance; apply nettle tea to skin, or use nettle cream or the homeopathic remedy for urticaria.
• Apis may also be used to treat rashes and inflammation associated with allergies.

ARTHRITIS AND RHEUMATISM
• Baths with apple cider vinegar are said to ease symptoms.
• Drink cleansing teas, such as burdock or sasaparilla, or warming teas, such as ginger or rosemary.
• Ginger compresses on the affected area will ease pain.

• Eucalyptus tea can be added to bathwater to soothe.
• Vinegar compresses can be applied to the affected joints to help shift any deposits.
• Drink infusions of meadowsweet daily.

ASTHMA
• Pine oil, which can be used in the bath or a vaporizer, will reduce incidence of attacks.
• Take Rescue Remedy when you feel asthma coming on, to ease symptoms and prevent it becoming a full-blown attack.
• A steam inhalation of chamomile, eucalyptus, or lavender essential oils can be taken during an attack and immediately afterwards, to ease panic and help to open airways.

BOILS AND ABSCESSES
• Apply a warm fig or honey poultice to the affected area.
• Soak a sterile cloth with hot thyme tea, and apply to the area.
• A hot cabbage leaf poultice, applied to the area, will help to draw out infection.

• Eat plenty of garlic if you are prone to boils. Garlic is cleansing, and chronic boils indicate that you may have a high number of toxins in your body.

• A warm compress with essential oil of chamomile, lemon, lavender, or thyme will help to bring the boil out.

• The homeopathic remedy Hepar Sulph may be helpful.

• Drink infusions of thyme or red clover three times daily during attacks.

• Drink echinacea two or three times daily to boost the immune system and purify the blood.

BRUISES

• Take the homeopathic remedy Arnica every three hours from the time of injury, to encourage healing. Tincture or cream can be applied to the affected area.

• Homeopathic remedy and tincture of Calendula will ease symptoms.

• Macerated and heated cabbage can be applied to the affected area.

• Use a mustard poultice to draw the blood away from the bruised area; black pepper oil will have the same effect.

• A vinegar compress can be used for all bruises or swelling. Avoid eye area.

• Witch hazel tincture can be used to relieve swellings and bruises. Apply as a cool compress.

• Use roasted onions in a poultice to help heal bruising.

COLDS

• Barley water with lemon and honey will encourage healing and shorten the duration of a cold.

• Cinnamon is an excellent warming herb, and can be added to food and drinks (and as an oil to a vaporizer) to treat and prevent colds and flu.

• Fresh garlic, eaten daily, will discourage the onset of a cold. Garlic will also work to reduce fever.

• Ginseng powder, added to any warming herbal tea, will boost the immune system and help the body to fight the infection.

• Honey, eaten fresh or added to herbal teas, will encourage healing and prevent secondary infections.

• Steep lemons in hot water and a little honey; drink regularly during a cold to restore, and prevent further infection. Will also treat coughs.

• Peppermint helps to reduce the symptoms of a cold.

• A mustard poultice on the chest, or mustard added to a footbath, will act as a decongestant.

• Citrus fruit is rich in vitamin C, which will help to fight infection.

• The herb echinacea will encourage the immune response, and acts as a natural antibiotic.

CONSTIPATION

• Apples are very cleansing, and will encourage bowel movements.

• Honey has laxative properties

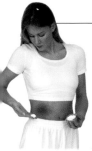

and can be added to food or drinks to relieve constipation. Try honey-bran muffins.

• Licorice is laxative; licorice tea, drunk before meals, will encourage the passing of stools.

• Strawberries, prunes, and spinach are laxative.

• Drink an infusion of elderflower or senna once daily, as needed.

• Make up a massage oil of black pepper, marjoram, and rosemary (one drop each in a light carrier oil), rub into the abdomen.

COUGHS

• Pine oil, in a vaporizer, will ease coughing and act to restore the lungs.

• A tincture of garlic (place several garlic cloves in brandy, and leave for two or three weeks, then strain) or garlic syrup (tincture, or fresh garlic mixed with a little honey) will help the body to fight infection. Ginseng in hot herbal tea warms the body and eases symptoms.

• Honey and lemon will ease coughs and encourage healing.

• Add slightly macerated licorice root sticks to herbal drinks, to ease coughing.

• Mustard powder, mixed with a little water, can be made into a poultice and applied to the chest area.

• A warm roasted onion poultice can also be applied to the chest. Drink warm onion broth to cleanse and reduce congestion.

• Peppermint tea can be drunk to soothe.

• Inhale essential oil of eucalyptus, which is expectorant and decongestant.

CYSTITIS

• Eat live yogurt, and use as a douche to ease the symptoms of cystitis, and prevent recurrence.

• Cranberry juice, drunk daily, will discourage bacteria from sticking to the walls of the bladder and urinary tract. It both treats and prevents the condition.

• Garlic tincture, added to food or warm drinks, will ease cystitis.

DIARRHEA

• Barley water will help to ease diarrhea.

• Limeflowers, drunk as a tea, will ease spasm, and soothe the digestive tract.

• Peppermint tea will treat diarrhea and other digestive problems.

• Ripe bananas can be eaten for diarrhea; they also help to build up the body's healthy bacteria, which will prevent further infection.

• Drink infusions of meadowsweet, golden seal, or slippery elm, up to three times daily as required.

• Slippery elm powder in a cup of hot water can be drunk three times daily, for all stomach and gastric upsets.

• Put one drop each of lavender, ginger, and orange oil in a few tablespoons of a light carrier oil. Massage into the abdominal area.

ECZEMA

• An oatmeal bath will soothe irritation and reduce itching.

• Internally, the following herbs may be useful. All of them have anti-inflammatory properties: chamomile, marigold, burdock, and red clover.

• Bathe the affected areas with a strong infusion of marigold.

• Chickweed ointment can be applied to areas of inflammation, pain, or itching, to ease symptoms.

• A gentle massage with a blend of chamomile, lavender, and/or Melissa in a little carrier oil can be used to treat eczema.

• Bathe sore patches with an infusion of witch hazel, diluted in some warm water.

• Massage the affected areas with essential oils of chamomile, sage, geranium, and lavender, all blended with a little carrier oil.

• See also allergies, page 53.

HEADACHES

• Place a dab of lavender oil on the nostrils to ease headaches. A lavender bath will have a similar effect.

• A ginger footbath may ease the pain, and warm the body.

• Chamomile tea is soothing, and will ease the symptoms.

• A tincture made from the fresh leaves of feverfew eases migraine. Combined with valerian, it is useful for migraine and other severe headaches caused by anxiety.

• The homeopathic remedy Coffea is beneficial for headaches caused by exhaustion from insomnia or from overstimulation.

• Inhale basil oil for migraine.

• Melissa in the bath or as a massage oil is uplifting and calming, both for migraine and other headaches.

• A mustard footbath is a traditional remedy for headaches.

• One of the following homeopathic remedies may be appropriate for persistent headaches: Belladonna, Bryonia, Gelsemium, Nux Vomica, or Pulsatilla.

• Mix lemon juice and bicarbonate of soda and warm water to ease headaches.

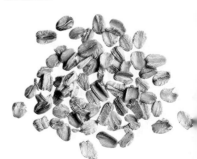

INDIGESTION

• Chamomile tea is a legendary digestive. Drink before meals and last thing at night to prevent heartburn and other digestive disorders.

• Fresh pineapple, eaten after a meal, will prevent attacks of indigestion.

• Clove tea and cinnamon tea are both digestive and will ease symptoms.

• Fresh dill, added to boiling water and steeped, will reduce flatulence and gas pains.

• Feverfew, eaten daily, will prevent migraine and reduce the incidence of headaches.

• Fennel – eaten raw or cooked, or bruised seeds infused, will act as a digestive.

• Chew ginger root for digestive disorders.

• Peppermint leaves can be infused and drunk to relieve indigestion, and to soothe any gas pains. Peppermint oil can be rubbed into the abdomen for instant relief.

• Drink a little warmed vinegar and honey in a cup of hot water to ease digestive complaints.

INSOMNIA

• Chamomile tea, drunk before bedtime, will encourage sleep.

• A few drops of lavender oil on the bedsheets or in a vaporizer by the bed, will help you to relax.

• The herbs valerian and vervain will aid relaxation.

• A number of Bach Flower Remedies will encourage sleep. Clematis might be useful, or vervain or Rescue Remedy, if it is difficult to relax. White Chestnut is suggested for mental activity which prevents sleep.

• Apply a chamomile compress to the head to encourage sleep.

• Clove and sage teas are both sedative.

• Lime flowers, skullcap, and borage are all soothing herbs and will assist sleep.

• Kali Phos, a homeopathic remedy, may be useful, or Coffea. Try Lycopodium if you are anxious, unable to get off to sleep, and then find it difficult to wake in the morning.

NAUSEA AND VOMITING

• Fennel or peppermint tea will ease nausea.

• Chew a ginger root to ease nausea.

• Clove or ginger tea can be used to ease the symptoms.

• Lavender will soothe and ease nausea.

• Peppermint eases nausea – particularly the nausea of travel sickness.

• Barley water may ease symptoms.

• Sip an infusion of cinnamon and meadowsweet until symptoms ease.

• Homeopathic remedies include: Nux Vomica, for nausea and vomiting after overeating or eating rich foods; Arsenicum for chilliness and diarrhea – often with food poisoning; Ipecacuanha, for a continuous feeling of nausea with pains in the stomach.

• Massage lemon essential oil into the abdomen (in a light carrier oil).

• Drink an infusion of lemon in warm water to cleanse and restore the digestive activity.

PERIOD PROBLEMS

• Drink carrot juice to prevent heavy periods.

• Cinnamon tincture may be added to a herbal drink to prevent heavy flow.

• Warm water with lemon juice will discourage heavy bleeding.

• The herb Agnus castus acts to balance hormones, working directly on the reproductive system. It is excellent for all "female" ailments.

• Hot fennel tea will encourage periods.

• Chamomile tea essential oil rubbed into the abdomen will reduce symptoms of painful periods.

• Peppermint tea will ease menstrual symptoms.

• Herbs that tone the uterus include raspberry leaf, cramp bark, and false unicorn root. Drink an infusion throughout the month.

• Herbs to relieve cramps include chamomile and valerian; drink an infusion or decoction two or three times daily, as needed.

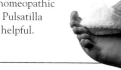

• The homeopathic remedy Mag Phos helps to reduce period pain.

THRUSH

• A live yogurt douche will encourage the growth of healthy bacteria (flora), which prevent fungal infection. Use regularly if you are prone to thrush.

• Apply yogurt to patches of oral thrush, and include live yogurt in your daily diet.

• Apple cider vinegar, added to warm water, can be used as a douche.

• Drink an infusion of echinacea or marigold to encourage healing, boost the immune system, and clear infection.

• A douche of marigold or lavender flowers will ease the symptoms of thrush.

• A tiny drop of tea tree oil, added to warm, previously boiled water, can be used as a douche.

• The homeopathic remedy Pulsatilla may be helpful.

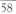

Further reading

Curtis, Susan; Fraser, Romy; and Kohler, Irene, NEAL'S YARD NATURAL REMEDIES (Arkana, 1988)

De Vries, Jan, TRADITIONAL HOME AND HERBAL REMEDIES (Mainstream Publishing, 1986)

Hoffman, David, THE COMPLETE ILLUSTRATED HOLISTIC HERBAL (Element, 1996)

Lawless, Julia, THE ILLUSTRATED ENCYCLOPEDIA OF ESSENTIAL OILS (Element, 1995)

McIntyre, Anne, HERBAL MEDICINE (Optima, 1987)

Sullivan, Karen (ed.), ILLUSTRATED ENCYCLOPEDIA OF NATURAL HOME REMEDIES (Element, 1997)

Useful addresses

AROMATHERAPY
International Federation of Aromatherapists
4 Eastmearn Road, London
SE21 8HA

FLOWER REMEDIES
Bach Flower Centre
Mount Vernon, Sotwell, Wallingford,
Oxfordshire OX10 0PZ

Dr. Edward Bach Healing Society
644 Merrick Road, Lynbrook
NY 11563 USA

HERBALISM
National Institute of Medical Herbalists
41 Hatherley Road, Winchester,
Hants SO22 6RR

California School of Herbal Studies
PO Box 39, Forestville,
CA 95436 USA

National Herbalists Association of Australia
14/249 Kingsgrove Road, Kingsgrove,
NSW 2208

HOMEOPATHY
Society of Homeopaths
2 Artizan Road, Northampton
NN1 4HU

National Center for Homeopathy
801 North Fairfax Street, Alexandra
VA 22314 USA

Australian Federation of Homeopaths
21 Bulah Close, Berowra Heights,
NSW 2082

OTHERS
Neal's Yard Agency
14 Neal's Yard, London WC2H 9DP
Free advice on therapies, workshops,
holidays and courses.
Neal's Yard Remedies 0181 879 0705